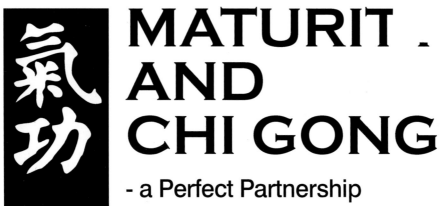

MATURIT
AND
CHI GONG

- a Perfect Partnership

By Peter Haines & Clive Birch

Maturity & Chi Gong - a Perfect Partnership

www.chi-gong.co.uk

ISBN 978-0-9541431-8-3

A catalogue record of this book is available from the British Library.

Printed and published by am-pm design & print, 35 Slaney Street, Gloucester, GL1 4TQ

Also by Peter Haines

**The Clarion Resource
A Matter of Public Interest
Priory**

And by Peter Haines and Clive Birch

So You Think We're Alone?

Further copies available from the publishers, 01452 332027, publishing@am-pm.co.uk.

Contents

Important Information

Every effort has been made to make the activities described in this book enjoyable, comfortable and, above all, safe.

Anyone in doubt about their physical fitness should consult their doctor before engaging in the activities described here.

The writers and publishers will not be held responsible in any way for any injury which may arise as a result of following the suggestions in this book.

Readers engaging in these activities do so entirely at their own risk.

Foreword

Maintaining our health and well-being as we mature is crucial to our quality of life in older age, both physically and mentally. For example, only one person in a group of seven fit and active older people will fall, but up to a third of older people say they limit their activity because of a fear of falling. This can have serious effects on a person's mobility and independence which can lead to a reduced quality of life and increase the risk of future falls. All of which can have an impact on family members and carers too.

We all have individual preferences as to how we can maintain our health and well-being, and the way that we can remain active changes over time. Gym sessions and Lycra, even if our scene in youth, may not appeal as we get older.

In maturity some people will maintain good levels of physical activity through a range of activities such as household chores, walking, gardening, sport or dancing whilst others with less mobility may also benefit from the gentle chair based and standing activities outlined here.

NHS Gloucestershire has been working with partner organisations for some time to develop a range of physical activity opportunities across the county to ensure that good levels of physical activity are achievable for everyone.

When we were approached by Clive last year, who has a wealth of experience in developing and delivering *tai chi* classes to all ages across Gloucestershire, his idea to produce a more accessible form of *tai chi – chi gong* - was something that we were keen to support. *Tai chi* is a form of exercise which already has evidence to show its effectiveness in improving balance and reducing the risk of falling, and this form of *tai chi* is suitable for a wide range of abilities.

The result has been true partnership working with Clive and Peter, the authors, and Martin and his team at 'am-pm publishing'.

This book and DVD will support and enhance the range of physical activity opportunities for older people across the county and can be used by individuals and groups alike. We hope that groups will enjoy getting together and having fun, using this book and DVD on a regular basis and, for some, following it up at home.

We are very pleased that Clive will be supporting the roll out of this publication across the county and if you are a member of a local group that would like to explore this opportunity, or other aspects of healthy active ageing, please contact us and we can arrange for a demonstration/visit as appropriate.

Dr Shona Arora
Joint Director Public Health
NHS Gloucestershire/ Gloucester County Council
February 2010

For further details contact Public Health Department on 08454 221500.

Acknowledgements

There are so many people to whom the authors are indebted; in fact, too many to be listed. However, special mention is necessary for those who have worked so hard to make this book and DVD possible and others who have contributed to knowledge, understanding and well-being. They include the team at NHS Gloucestershire, Fu Yi, Bruce Frantzis, Ko Hung, Master Lam, Barbara Piranty, Daniel Reid and Dr Yang Jwing-Ming. We also make special mention of Martin Seccombe of am-pm publishing without whose patience and tolerance this book would never have reached you.

And to those whose name should appear here but does not, we apologise in the hope you will forgive and understand our omission due to space and poor recall.

Preface

Clive Birch has developed these exercises and routines over a number of years. Specifically they were designed to assist the more mature among us who suffer some of the ailments we so often put down to normal ageing. Much of his work has been done in classes and nursing homes with the chair bound, those who experience difficulties with their mobility, and some who are prone to falls.

And which of us who no longer looks forward to our next birthday, would welcome an improvement in our eyesight? Well, me for one.

We're all different and react differently and must expect different outcomes. Nevertheless, by practising just a little *chi gong* each day, it will be a rare person who experiences no mobility, flexibility or emotional improvement at all.

Based on the ancient art of *chi gong*, a form of *tai chi*, these exercises are simple, gentle and hopefully enjoyable. Some of the exercises in *Maturity & Chi Gong - a Perfect Partnership* originate from sources other than *chi gong*. These are mentioned at the appropriate point.

Introduction

As life moves on and the years pass by, unless we are conscious of our body and its requirements, the tendency in Western countries is to accept increasing limitations. We put on weight, the body stiffens and our bones lose density. To add to all that, our balance deteriorates. This can lead to falls which further weakens our bodies. We say to those around us, "It's age, it's inevitable. I can't do what I used to do." Anyone recognise this?

This attitude is entirely unnecessary. We do not need to physically age in the way we think we do. Maybe our culture has misled us? People in the 'less civilised' East, particularly China, have a different perspective. Certainly those who practise the techniques that we describe in *Maturity & Chi Gong - a Perfect Partnership* have a very different perspective on ageing.

Let's start with a few success stories. When Clive moved into his forties he started to become arthritic in two fingers. One of them had been damaged in childhood and was misshapen from that ancient accident. Naturally enough, being from a Western culture, he shrugged his shoulders putting the arthritis down to inevitability, and got on with his life. After he found *chi gong* and started practising regularly for a couple of years, he realised that the arthritis had disappeared. He hadn't worked on his fingers especially. In fact he had forgotten all about them. So not only was the outcome of *chi gong* a success in slowing down his ageing processes, but it also reversed the damage and ageing in his fingers. You can imagine the impact this had on his morale and his determination to continue to practise and explore these techniques.

The man who taught Clive many of the routines he learned in the first two years of *chi gong* was extremely sprightly and energetic. He was not keen on telling Clive his age. One day however, he let slip an incident in his young manhood that had occurred sixty years before. By working back, Clive realised that his teacher was now in his eighties. This was a man who was teaching *chi gong* to forty students each week. How many people in their eighties do you know who are teaching to that degree? Probably not many.

There was a reason why Clive started working with this venerable gentleman rather than other *chi gong* teachers. He discovered that this Englishman was teaching an Oriental discipline to Oriental students; this was despite there being Oriental teachers locally. These students knew they were onto a good thing. Soon after starting his lessons, Clive realised that it was to his considerable benefit he'd placed his learning in this teacher's charge.

In recent times a master of *chi gong* died in China… she was 104 years old. Now, the key point for Clive was not that she had lived to such a great age, but that she was teaching to within weeks of her death. Thus it dawned on Clive that not only does regular, assiduous practise of *chi gong* assist in extending normal lifespan, but it also collapses the physical decline period. Of course, the government and the pension funds might not be overjoyed if too many of us extended our lifetimes too far beyond the allotted three score and ten. The paying out from beleaguered pension schemes that are already crumbling at the edges would be a real headache. The newly invigorated mature people would be running around having fun for forty plus years after official retirement! So it seems unlikely that we'll find pension funds support for the techniques that are presented in *Maturity & Chi Gong - a Perfect Partnership*. Nevertheless these techniques have the potential to extend your life and, most importantly, enhance the quality of your life, when practised regularly.

Chi gong practitioners say that *chi* can be explained as an energy form, similar to electricity, which flows through human and animal bodies. When this circulation becomes stagnant or stops, the person or animal becomes sick or dies.

Chi is circulated and distributed through the body via channels called meridians; a network of major and minor channels which form a complex grid. These are found adjacent to nerve fibres and arteries, according to Dr Yang Jwing-Ming. The grid serves both the circulatory and nervous systems. *Chi* circulates through the body continuously.

Chi gong blends soft, gentle movements of the body with a calm contemplative state of mind.

Who is going to benefit?

Chi gong can benefit absolutely anyone, but we've designed the exercises in this book especially to help people with issues and conditions they would prefer to be without. Again we say, few people will find no benefit from *Maturity & Chi Gong - a Perfect Partnership*.

Those who prefer gentle exercise will enjoy *chi gong*. Mature people will love this journey of discovery, and maybe some of the young ones will as well. Clive has worked with people from 13 to 103 and all ages in between.

At each new class, Clive introduces his students to his two objectives. They are clear and uncompromising. He aims to work with every student to achieve two things; first to keep them out of the doctor's surgery, and second, to keep people in their homes for as long as possible.

So, for all of you who wish to do something about the following, we wish you well and are confident you'll derive benefit from the exercises. As we've said, remember we're all different, react differently and can expect different outcomes. But with a little patience, most people will find improvements; some small, some dramatic.

- **Mobility problems.** Frustration and inconvenience result if we are unable to get about and do those things we want to do.

- **Confidence.** Feel better about ourselves and the way we are. Most of us experience times in our lives when we feel negative about ourselves. And how debilitating that can be. Our confidence affects so much of the way we perform in so many activities and environments. Notice those who you perceive as being self-confident. (OK, they may be acting, but it may also be that they are truly confident.) Notice also it is they who seem to succeed so often. How come then, that we can't do likewise? Well, we can, you know? We really can, with just a little time and effort put into the exercises here.

- **Dexterity.** With the exercises described and demonstrated in *Maturity & Chi Gong - a Perfect Partnership*, we will feel more in control of our bodies. That's good news for all of us who feel we are suffering from the ageing process. Of course we tend to lose our dexterity as the years roll by; but it's not inevitable.

  Remember Clive damaged the fourth finger of his right hand in his youth. More than 50 years later, the finger seized up completely. In no way improving matters, the adjacent third finger joined it, becoming stiffer and stiffer. Now he had two useless fingers. He started *chi gong* and it was two years later that he realised that both fingers were back to normal... totally mobile.

- **Balance.** When our physical balance improves, so does our psychological balance and in turn our confidence grows. The prevention of falls is important to us all. Improved balance will contribute to reducing the risk of falls.

- **Eyesight.** This is so important to all of us as it impacts upon everything we do and much of what we are. Yet we can improve our eyesight, believe it or believe it not. That's why there's a special exercise devoted to eyesight (Section Four).

But while these exercises would benefit just about anyone, one way or another, that doesn't mean they are suitable for everyone. Those of us with a more impatient, impetuous nature might well become bored quickly before the positive results become apparent.

How to use Maturity & Chi Gong - a Perfect Partnership

The choice is yours of course, but it is recommended you work through *Maturity & Chi Gong - a Perfect Partnership* section by section. Repeat the exercises until you're happy and comfortable with them. The system is flexible however. If you wish to go to the standing exercises first then, by all means, do so.

You might choose to use this book by itself, or with support of the DVD. You might even choose to use just the DVD. Whichever you choose, remember to have fun.

Section One is designed to help those with mobility problems. All the exercises are completed while seated. You will discover that the exercises in Sections One and Two are completed seated. There is good reason for this. Physical stablity and falls prevention are improved when whole body flexibility is improved. *Chi gong* is holistic.

Most of the seated exercises can be performed standing. It is best to be patient when extending the range of exercises that you wish to work with. When you are confident and feel ready, add seated exercises gradually and perform them standing.

But before you do the seated exercises standing, please ensure you have gained your confidence with the exercises in Section Three.

Section Two contains enhanced exercises to complement Section One.

Section Three has several standing routines. Some people with mobility problems may not be able to do these exercises. But for those who can it's important to work through them. They will improve your mobility.

Section Four contains an eye exercise. Eyes use a lot of energy.

Remember improved FLEXIBILITY leads to BETTER POSTURE leads to CONFIDENCE leads to GREATER PHYSICAL STRENGTH leads to IMPROVED STANDING, WALKING and FALLS PREVENTION.

A short history of chi gong

The true roots of *chi gong* are lost in the mists of time. Master Lam says that the study of human energy, the Chinese call this *chi*, can be traced back to the reign of the Yellow Emperor, thought to be around 2690-2590 BC. He is said to have practised *chi gong* techniques and lived to a ripe old age of 111 years, despite the distraction of his harem of 1,200 women!

Daniel Reid claims that *chi gong* first took root in prehistoric times in ancient China, around 10,000 years ago, with a ceremonial dance known as the 'Great Dance'. This was found to have therapeutic consequences for those who practised it. Medicine and *chi gong* were the preserve of tribal shamans whose role it was to commune with the powers of Heaven and Earth.

The first written references to *chi gong*, again according to Daniel Reid, are found in texts 4,000 years old. One dance was specifically developed to ward off disease, regulate breathing, and balance energy in the damp atmosphere of the Yellow River Basin where Chinese civilisation developed.

Other sources say that the ancient Chinese saw that animals didn't suffer from the same degenerative diseases with which people were so troubled. They began to practise the animal movements. Lo and behold, assiduous practise eliminated these degenerative diseases and *chi gong* was born.

Nearly 2,000 years ago, the scholar Fu Yi wrote, "*Chi gong* is an art that pleases the spirit, slows the ageing process and prolongs life." Daniel Reid tells us that archaeological evidence, unearthed at Ma Wang tombs in Hunan Province, has shown that *chi gong* was widely practised in the Han period nearly 2,000 years ago. They are still in use today. Documents, scrolls and anatomical charts, with detailed diagrams of the human energy system, show *chi gong* movement and breathing systems. These discoveries provided proof that by the second century AD, the internal school of energy cultivation had supplanted the external school of toxic mineral compounds. This then, provided the basis for the development of human longevity and that this could only be achieved through disciplined practise.

In the fourth century AD, Taoist philosopher Ko Hung wrote a treatise 'He who Embraces the Uncarved Block'. In this he claimed that by cultivating internal energy, one could live a long and healthy life. In so doing, practitioners would gain sufficient time and energy to lay the foundation for immortal existence in the spiritual world, after the death of the body. Towards the end of the Ching dynasty in 1912 AD, the walls of secrecy that retained *chi gong* secrets within the *lineage families*, began to crumble. Total disintegration came with the end of the Civil War in 1949.

It is interesting that *chi gong*, the alleged root of all *tai chi* and martial art systems, came to the West and has started to make its presence felt here. It is really only in the past decade that it has become popular. Now its popularity grows daily along with a respect for its efficacy. Bruce Frantzis, an American who lived in the East for twenty years, became a *lineage master* after working with the previous lineage holder in China. He has a story to tell. Prior to the end of the Chinese Civil War in 1949, most of the knowledge concerning *chi gong* was held in secret by certain families (lineage families) in China. In this way they could maintain their power and authority, particularly healing power, over others.

At the end of the Civil War when the communists came to power, the health system in the country collapsed. Many doctors and nurses were dead and hospitals had been destroyed. Mao Tse-Tung, the new leader of China, went to the families who held the *chi gong* knowledge and asked them to release it for the benefit of the masses. The families refused. Mao responded with an ultimatum.

"Unless you release the knowledge that you hold concerning the healing properties of *chi gong*, I will kill everyone in your family; men, women, children, relatives near and far, everyone."

The families caved in and the knowledge was released, so much so that *chi gong* departments were started in hospitals, particularly military hospitals.

Mao was quoted as saying that Chinese civilisation's two greatest gifts to the world would prove to be Chinese food and Chinese medicine. He may yet prove to be correct.

Chi gong was unknown in the West until President Nixon visited China in 1973. At that time this ancient culture opened its knowledge to outsiders. Some Chinese emigrated to the West, particularly the USA, where techniques were taught and books were written.

Despite its age, the study of *chi* remains an active field of research, continuing in China and other parts of the world.

Chi gong and its relevance to us today

"So what does all this *chi gong* stuff have to do with me?" we hear you cry. Well, absolutely nothing for those who have no interest in their vitality, mobility, eyesight and quality of life, except perhaps as academic interest. However, if you are interested in addressing some of those life issues, then open your minds and have a go. After all, there's not much you can lose other than a little time and the price of *Maturity & Chi Gong - a Perfect Partnership*. And who knows, you might find it works and you might even discover you have had some fun along the way.

There are some 200 million people out there today who have discovered *chi gong*. Once they were just like the rest of us. Each of them had to have started *chi gong* at some point, but start they did. And were they glad? Well, after you've read a little more and practised some of the exercises, decide that for yourself.

Let's see what *chi gong* and the exercises in this book can do for you.

If you choose to develop your skills further, there is likely to be a class near you. But please remember; don't rush it. Don't go too fast without help, support and guidance. Some of the more advanced exercises carry a risk if they are not attempted properly under the guidance of a skilled practitioner.

What others say

That's quite enough words from us for now. Let's hear what others have said about *chi gong*. Clive's own students make wonderful advocates for the exercises in *Maturity & Chi Gong - a Perfect Partnership*.

I would love to make some comments on the chi gong. I think the exercises are very gentle but very effective, especially for people who are disabled or restricted in their movements. There's a nice feeling of having worked out, but also of feeling relaxed. I think it also helps with self esteem and feeling good about yourself. Finally, the exercises are done very slowly and safely. I hope these comments are helpful, as I personally enjoyed the classes very much.
Julia is recovering from a stroke and says, "Now I live life to the full."

It is energising. I feel good after it. **Jenny Jay.**

It is a great confidence builder. **Kathy Hector.**

There are strong physiological reasons for chi gong. The musculature actions in chi gong stimulate the lymphatic system positively. The lymphatic has been undersold as an important generator of health to the general public. **Peter Jay, 'A' level biology teacher.**

It works every part of the body, all the muscle groups, relaxing and strengthening at the same time. You find out for yourself what your body is capable of and it is great fun. **Jan Ferguson.**

I have found chi gong to be particularly beneficial in the case of arthritis and ME. The exercises energise and enliven a sluggish system and stiff painful limbs at the same time as creating a sense of inner peace, balance and well-being. **Mary Fitzgerald.**

It is very peaceful and spiritual for me especially with music. **Joan Fitzgerald.**

Mature students' first experience of chi gong

In the summer of 2005 a 6 week pilot scheme introducing mature people to the benefits of *chi gong* was funded by Cotswold and Vale Primary Care Trust. From day centres and older people's groups, 80 people took part, all from the county of Gloucestershire.

Ages of participants ranged from 61 to 94 (the average age was 80). Many had only limited mobility and some 60% had indicated that they had a long-term ailment or illness. Arthritis was the most common ailment. Other complaints included osteoporosis, asthma, high blood pressure, Parkinson's and the after effects of stroke. Hip replacements, high blood pressure, diabetes and lymphoedema were also cited.

Half of the day centre respondents had participated in physical activity in the previous 12 months; mainly walking or "general exercises". Over one third of the older people's group members had taken part in activity similar to *chi gong*; mainly yoga.

> Prior to the pilot, participants were asked what they hoped to gain from it. They cited
> - Flexibility/suppleness/loosen joints/movement in joints
> - To help back/hip/knee
> - Improve fitness/general exercise
> - To improve general health
> - Well-being/to feel better
> - Relaxation
> - Curiosity/out of interest/to try something new.

These seem to be as good reasons as any to try *chi gong*.

After the six week programme of *chi gong*, half (49%) the day care respondents had noticed improvements and over 80% made positive comments. On the other hand, no participants made negative comments. The following results were cited; improved circulation, reduced stiffness, improved mobility, improved strength, better breathing, more energy, feeling of well-being, more relaxed and more active.

One day centre manager said all her participants wanted her to convey how impressed they were with their tutor; one Clive Birch.

From the older persons' groups, more than 75% indicated they had experienced improvements including being more relaxed, more flexible, more lively, feeling fitter, improved breathing and feeling more positive. In all, 80% said they would like to continue with *chi gong*.

Our thanks to Barbara Piranty and Gloucestershire Rural Community Council for allowing us to reproduce these research findings.

Let's get started

Let's start by preparing your environment. Find somewhere that is not cold, but is calm and quiet. Try to avoid bright and aggressive colours; reds and oranges. They detract from the subtle process. Try to ensure you have sufficient personal space. Strip lighting is not advised. It isn't conducive to this gentle art, perhaps because of the flashing?

That's dealt with the environment, now think about what to wear. There are no hard and fast rules, but there is no reason not to feel comfortable. Try loose clothing, soft shoes or bare feet. Soon your choice of clothing will become second nature. You'll know what's best for you.

Last but not least, there's your state of mind to consider. Open mindedness is always a virtue in so many aspects of our lives, no less so than with the exercises we work through together in *Maturity & Chi Gong - a Perfect Partnership*. Those of you who are prepared to try something new will find adapting to these exercises easier than those who are resistant by nature. Patient people will enjoy the results more quickly than others.

Having said all this, nothing mentioned here is an essential ingredient for success. They are merely suggestions to help you, to make your experience more pleasurable and possibly speed up the positive results.

Now it's time for you to have some fun.

Section One
Mobility and General Health

As we get older, we in the West expect the ageing experience to become more and more painful. That's a miserable prospect, but it needn't be that way for all of us. In the East there are those with a very different attitude towards the inevitability of unpleasant consequences of ageing... those who regularly practise *chi gong*.

These are not muscle building exercises, although they will help to keep yours healthy and develop a toned body. They work with the internal energies generated through meridians and acupuncture points.

In Section One we will explore a daily routine that can form the basis for your improved health. Later on we'll show you some additional elements that you'll find helpful.

All the exercises in Section One are performed from the sitting position. Make yourself comfortable in a straight back chair. Place both feet flat on the floor.

In *chi gong* concentration is the key to success. Everything is controlled by the mind.

Try to do as many exercises as you can. Don't worry if you can't do them all to begin with. With just a little practise you soon find yourself completing them. Concentrate on relaxation, slow, regular movements without strain. Try to make it an enjoyable experience.

1.1 Head Turns

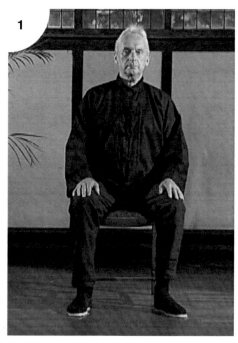

Sit upright, head up, neck straight, and relax your shoulders.

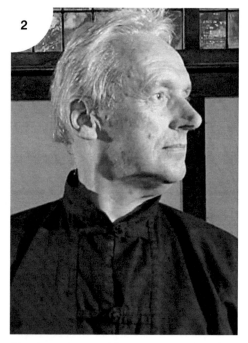

Slowly and smoothly move your head to the left, at the same time breathe in. Turn as far as is comfortable then slowly and smoothly, move your head back to the centre, breathing out at the same time. Breath in as you turn, breathe out as you return.

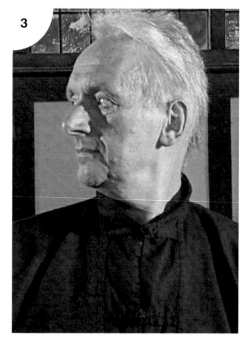

Stop briefly in the middle and slowly and smoothly move your head to the right, at the same time breathe in. Turn as far as is comfortable.

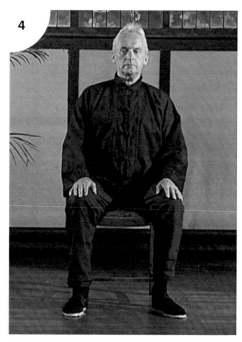

Now move your head back to the centre slowly and smoothly, breathing out at the same time.

Repeat the whole cycle a number of times. The number of repeats can be increased over time as you become more mobile.

22

1.2 Head Forward and Back

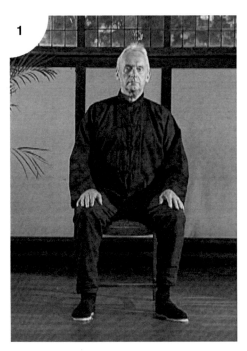

Sit upright with your head up, neck straight and shoulders relaxed.

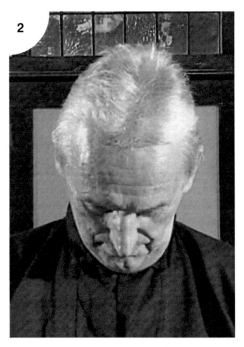

Drop your head and chin towards your chest.

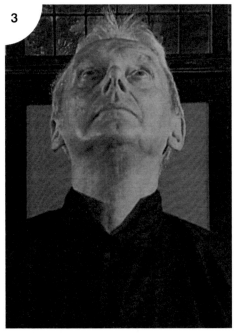

Slowly, smoothly and rhythmically move your head back so your chin points towards the ceiling and back again to your chest. Be careful not to go back too far as that will compress the spine.

Repeat this a number of times.

1.3 Head Circles

This third neck exercise is more demanding than the first two, and should only be attempted after the first two have been completed. Your neck will have been stretched and warmed up by then.

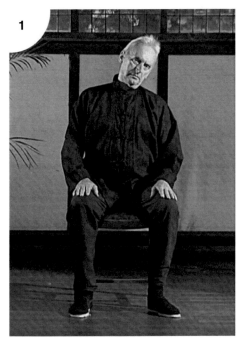

Gently lower your head to one side so that your ear is as close to your shoulder as possible.

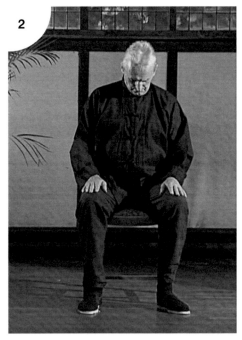

Slowly and rhythmically drop your head round to the front of your chest in a semi-circular motion until the opposite ear is as close as is comfortable to the other shoulder.

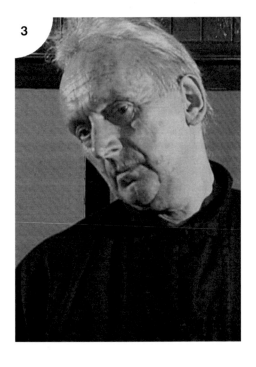

Repeat in the other direction. Try this a few more times but only for as long as it's comfortable.

1.4 Cruncher

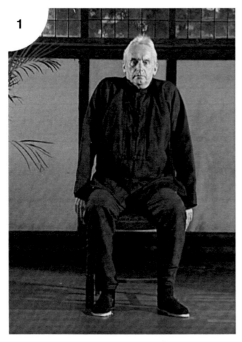

Keeping your neck and arms relaxed, raise both shoulders in the direction of your ears.

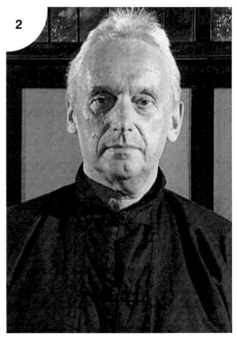

Relax and drop them back to their normal position.

Repeat this a number of times and you'll benefit from the alternate stressing and relaxing motion. This alternating stressing and relaxing causes blood to rush into your shoulders and neck, bringing energy with it. This is the energy that the Chinese call chi.

1.5 Shoulder Rotation

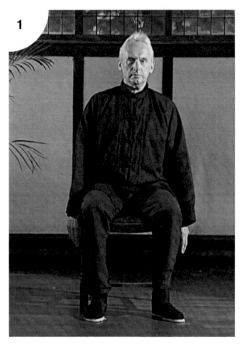

Relax both arms down by your sides.

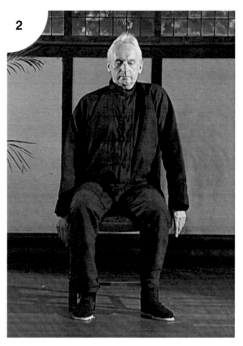

Very slowly rotate one shoulder in a circle. As you do this relax your arm, hand and neck. Complete 4 to 6 circles then move the shoulder in the opposite direction.

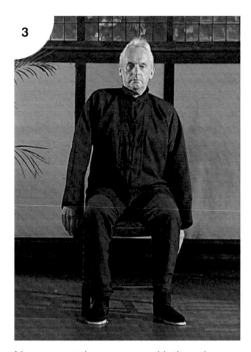

Now repeat the process with the other shoulder.

1.6 Hand Press 1

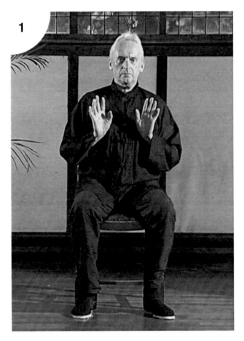

Place both hands, palms out, with the backs as close to your chest as possible.

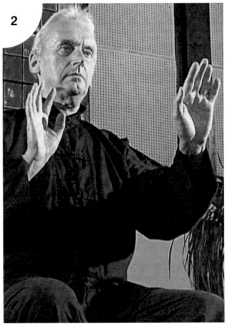

Move one arm out slowly and rhythmically and stop before your elbow straightens.

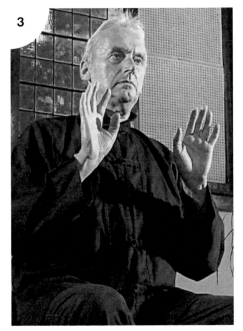

Bring your arm back to its starting position.

Repeat 8 or 10 times with each arm.

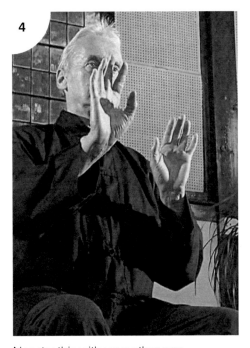

Now try this with your other arm.

All movements should be completed slowly and rhythmically. This simple exercise is extremely beneficial in maintaining blood flow along your arms, right to your fingers.

1.7 Hand Press 2

This is a development of Hand Press 1.

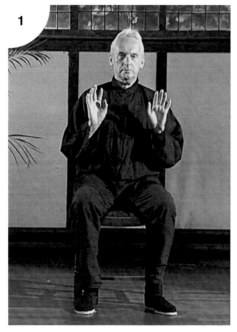

Place both hands, palms out, in front of your chest, just like Exercise 1.6.

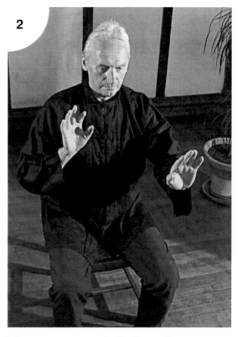

Move one arm out slowly and rhythmically, stopping before the elbow straightens.

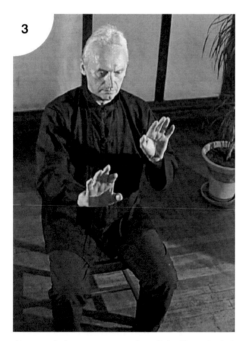

As you bring your arm back to the start position, move the other arm out at the same time.
Now both your arms are alternately moving backwards and forwards.
Repeat this 8 or 10 times.

This is an excellent exercise to improve the integration of both hemispheres of the brain.

1.8 Circle the Lower Arms

(Rather wickedly called the "Royal Wave" by Clive.)

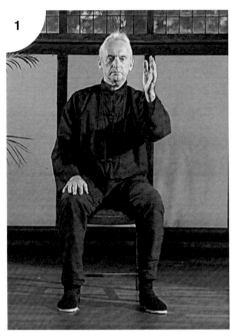

Hold one arm out in front of you. Release your armpit keeping it unrestricted. Be sure it's relaxed and your elbow bent.

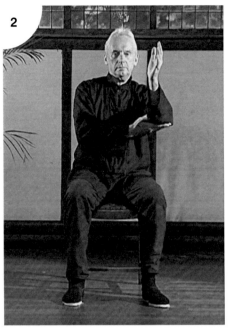

Support the elbow with the palm of the other hand.

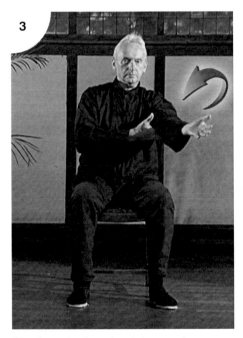

Slowly and relaxed, rotate your lower arm retaining the bend at your elbow.

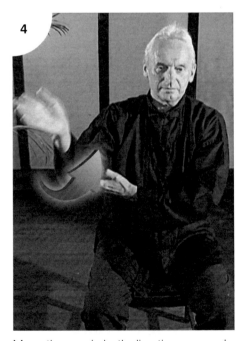

Move the arm in both directions several times. Now repeat with the other arm.

This exercise will improve mobility in your elbows.

1.9 Double Circle Arms

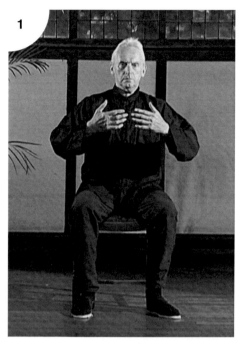

Hold both arms out in front of you. Don't close your armpit by pulling it close into your body; leave it loose. Keep your elbows bent and palms towards you as if clasping a beach ball to your chest. Your hands will be parallel to the floor but your elbows will be slightly lower.

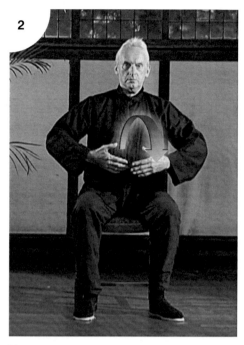

Move both arms out together describing a circle, and then back and up towards your chest.

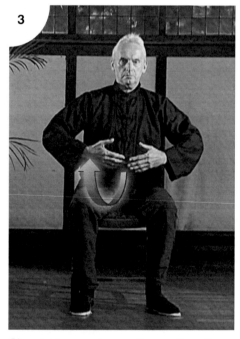

Change the rotation and move the other way. Repeat both movements 6 times.

1.10a Loosening the Shoulders

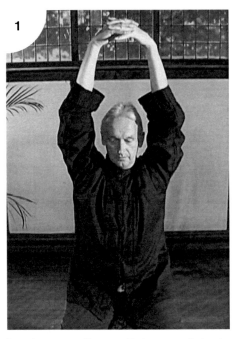

Interlace your fingers. Raise your linked hands above your head.

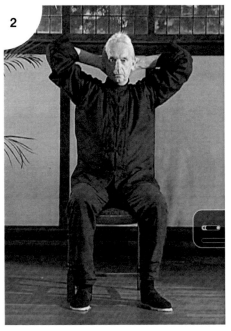

Drop your hands so your palms rest on your neck. If your hands can't go all the way down to your neck, then take the movement as far as you can.

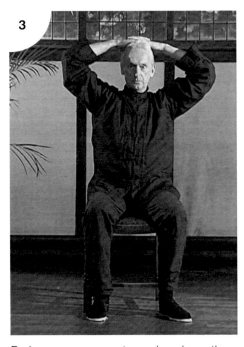

Perhaps you can rest your hands on the top of your head.

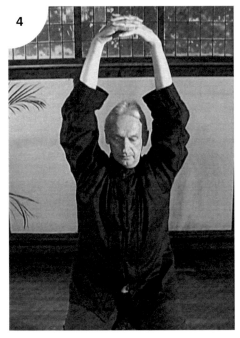

Return your hands above your head. Repeat this several times.

This is a great exercise after a long drive. It loosens the top of your spine and your shoulders. Try it.

1.10b Loosening the Shoulders

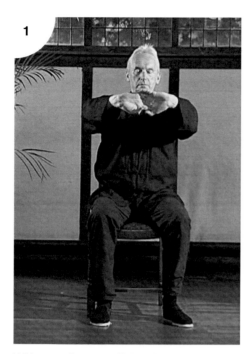

1

With your fingers still interlaced, gently and slowly push both hands out in front of your chest; palms out.

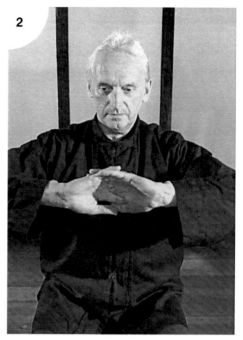

2

Now bring your hands back to your chest. Don't straighten your elbows. Repeat the whole process a number of times.

This exercise works the muscles at the top of your back and the top of your spine.

1.11 Finger Exercise 1

This exercise is taken from the Tibetan movement system, Seamm Jasani. This is a gentle way of starting the hand exercises and is especially useful for those with very stiff fingers.

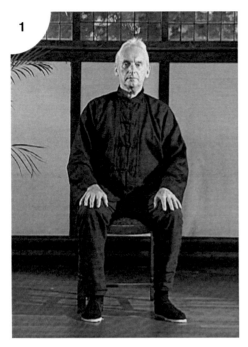

Place both palms on your knees.

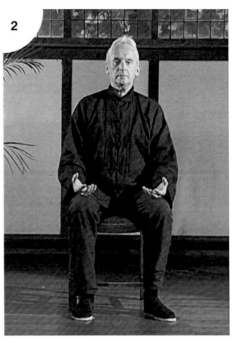

Turn your hands over so the palms are facing up. Curl your fingers as if you were holding a tennis ball. Hold this position for about 30 seconds.

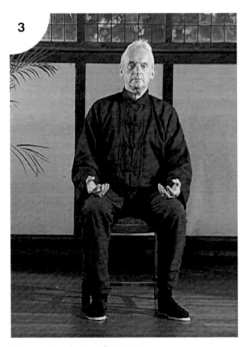

Now uncurl your fingers.

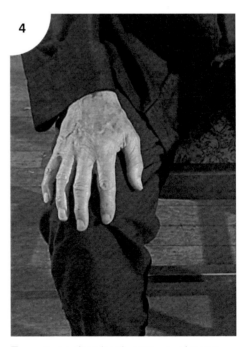

Turn your palms back onto your knees. Repeat exercises twice more.

1.12 Finger Exercise 2

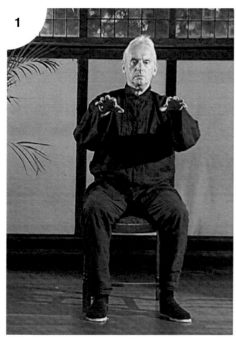

With palms facing downwards, raise both your hands in front of your chest.

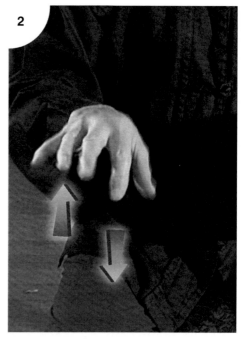

Move all your fingers up and down as vigorously and rhythmically as you are able, perhaps a little like playing a piano. Keep your hands and arms steady. Do as much as possible without straining.

This is excellent for relieving stiffness and helping with arthritic and rheumatic aches and pains.

1.13 Hand Exercise

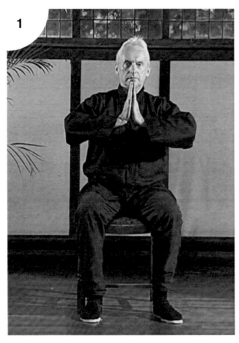

1

Press your hands together in front of your chest, similar to the prayer position.

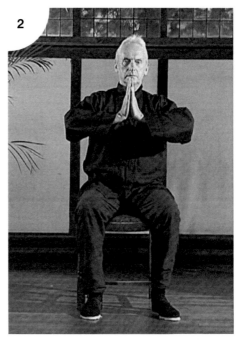

2

Raise your lower arms so they're parallel to the floor. Don't worry if you can't get your arms quite there. Just raise them as far up as you can.

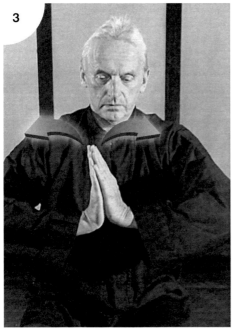

3

Use each hand in turn to press the fingers of your other hand back. Keep your elbows up if you can. Press just as hard as is comfortable.

Regular use of this exercise will improve mobility in your wrists and strengthen your grip.

1.14 Finger Exercise 3

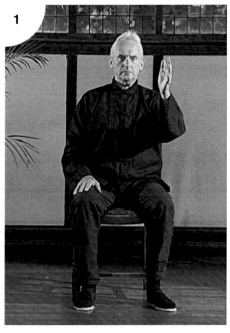

Hold one arm out in front of your body, making sure your elbow is bent.

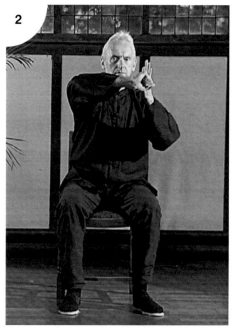

Wrap the palm of the other hand around the little finger and pull outwards and away from you, releasing as you do so. Try to be gentle but firm.

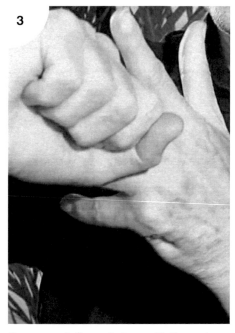

Grasp each finger in turn with the palm of the other hand.

4

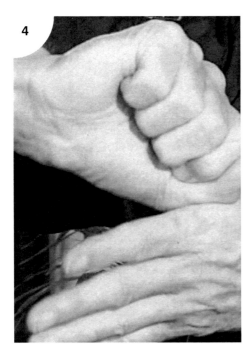

Pull each finger outwards without exerting any excess strain.

5

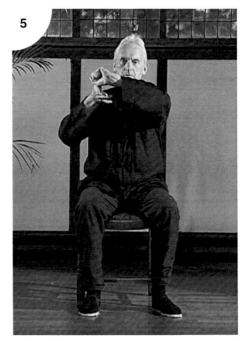

Now switch to your other hand.

When you are comfortable with this exercise you can repeat it several times. This exercise aids flexibility in the joints and fingers.

1.15 Turning the Waist

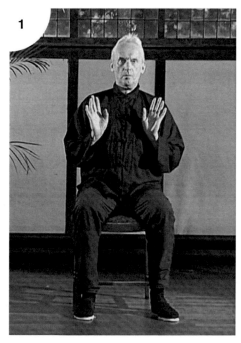

Bring both hands up to your chest, palms facing away from you.

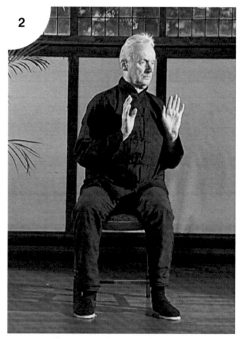

Turn your body SLOWLY from the waist, first to the left. Keep your torso straight, making the movement with conscious thought. Ensure that the turn is from your waist and NOT your neck or shoulders. Only turn as far as is comfortable.

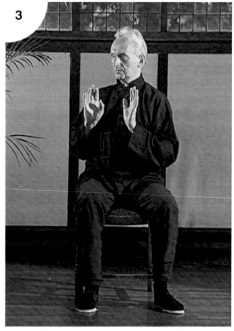

Now turn to the right. Repeat this exercise a number of times.

This helps with your flexibility.

1.16 Foot Rotation

Remember you're still sitting. Try this with your shoes on or off, whichever suits you best.
This exercise is best performed slowly and rhythmically to derive the most benefit. It isn't easy though.
If you find this difficult initially, please don't worry. With practise you'll find it becomes easier.

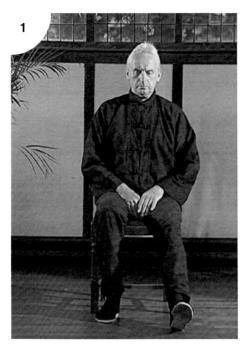

Bring one foot out in front.

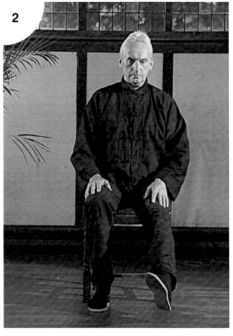

Either lift your foot off the ground or rest your heel on the floor.

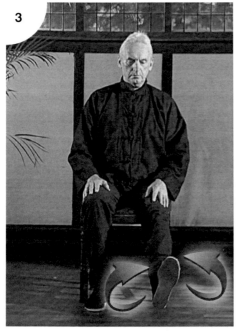

Rotate your ankle slowly. Make a number of rotations, left and right, as many times as feels comfortable.

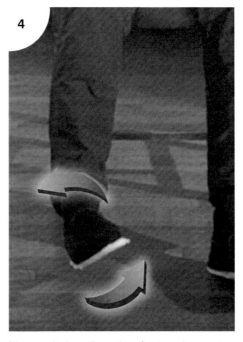

Now switch to the other foot and repeat the exercise.

1.17 Ankle Stretch

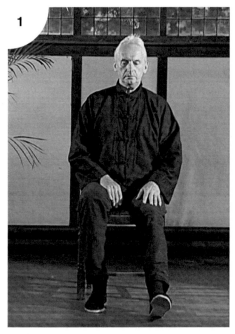

As with Exercise 1.16, bring one foot out in front and either lift the foot or rest your heel on the floor. Apart from your foot, keep the remainder of your leg steady, eliminating as much movement as possible.

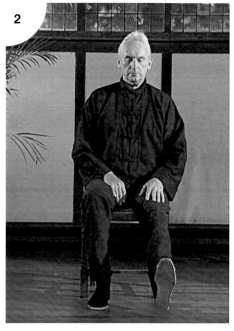

Bring your foot towards you then relax it.

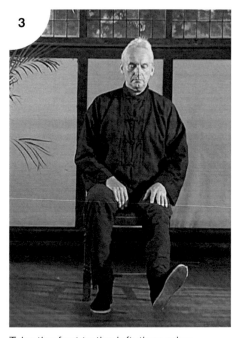

Take the foot to the left, then relax.

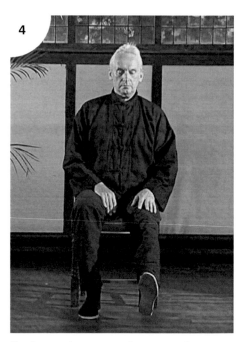

Push your toes away from you, then relax.

5

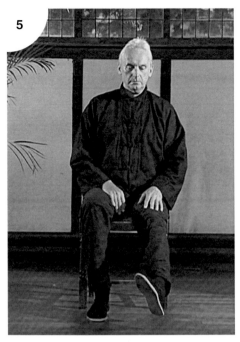

Now take the foot to the right, then relax.

6

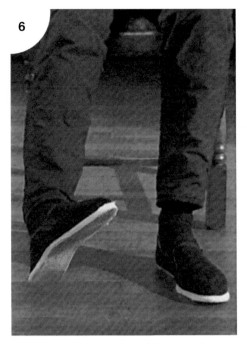

Now repeat the routine with your other foot. Relax the foot at the end. Repeat the whole routine as many times as is comfortable. Don't overdo it.

1.18 Toe Stretch

You may find it beneficial to remove your shoes for this exercise. Maybe you have already? Good. This helps the circulation as do Exercises 1.16 and 1.17 above.

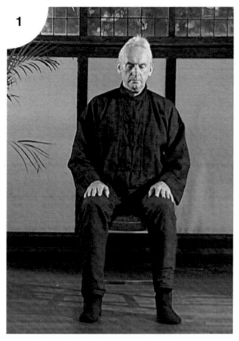

Place both your feet flat on the floor.

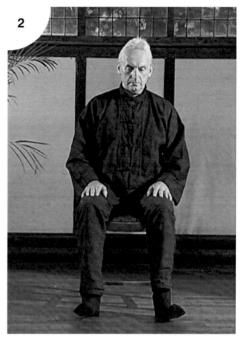

Keeping your feet and legs relaxed, stretch your toes out. Hold this for a few seconds and then relax them.

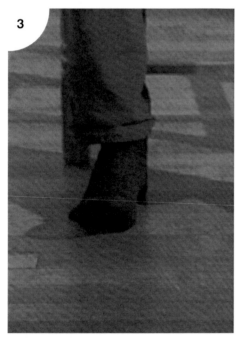

Stretch and relax, stretch and relax.
Repeat as many times as is comfortable.

This helps with circulation.

1.19 Knee Energising

This strengthens the meridian energy constantly exiting from the acupuncture points in the centre of your palms.

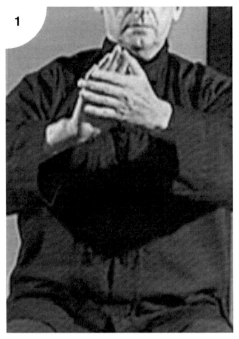

Rub the palms of your two hands together for a minute.

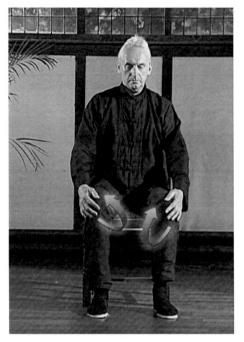

Now place both palms on the outside of each knee. Slowly rotate the palms around both knees from the outside in. Repeat this 12 times or as many times as are comfortable.

This energises the knees and is self nurturing. (Makes you feel good about yourself. Try it, and see.)

1.20 Knee Rotation

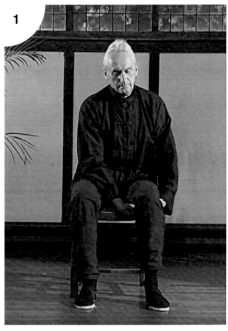

Interlace your fingers and support one leg with both hands by cradling your leg just above the knee.

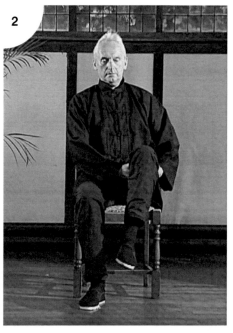

Lift the leg.

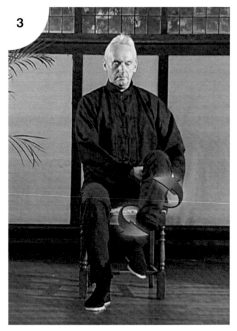

Rotate the knee several times both ways. Keep your lower leg and ankle particularly relaxed. Try this at least four times each way.

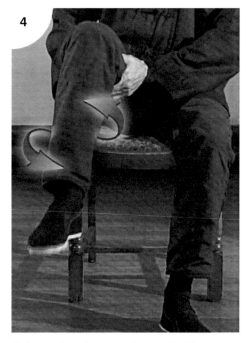

Put your leg down and repeat with your other leg. Again keep your ankle and foot relaxed.

1.21 Breathing Exercise

It is important to breathe gently. What is breathed in is not just air but cosmic energy, and forceful breathing will constrict the flow of cosmic energy. Check that your whole body is relaxed.

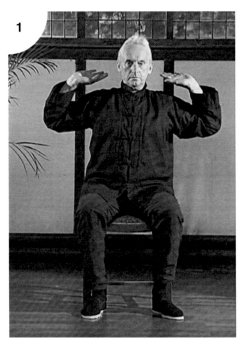

Place both hands above your shoulders with the palms up and elbows out. Breathe in through the nose.

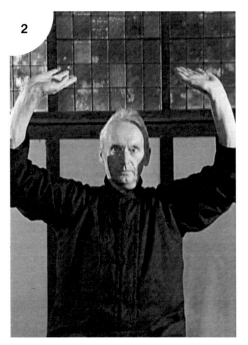

Push up with both hands at the same time, breathing out through the mouth as slowly and rhythmically as is comfortable.

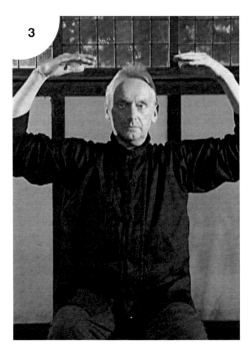

Turn your palms over and bring your hands back towards your shoulders breathing in again slowly and rhythmically. Repeat this a number of times.

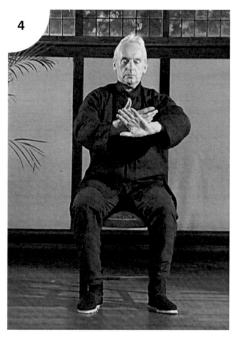

4

For the second part of this exercise, bring both hands down in front of your chest. The backs of your hands should be together with the left palm facing out and the right palm facing towards you.

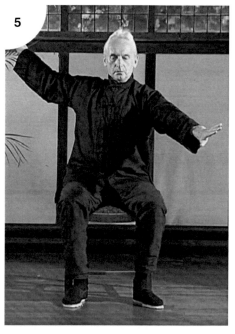

5

Move both hands away from each other while breathing in through the nose.

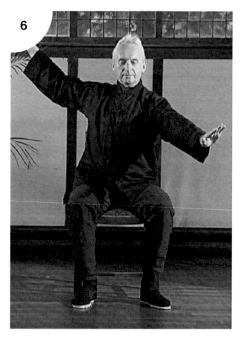

6

Stretch your right arm behind and back as far as is comfortable. Stretch your left arm away from you as far as is comfortable. This is one continuous movement.

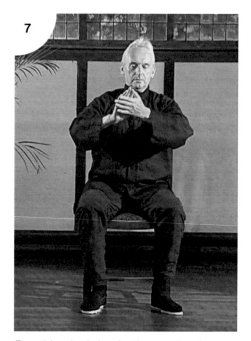

7

Breathing in, bring both arms back towards each other turning the left wrist until the palms of the hands touch.

8

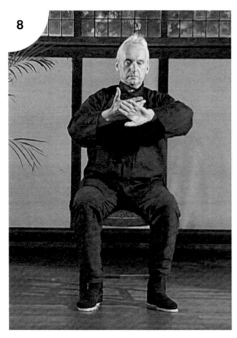

Turn your left hand so the backs of your hands are together again.
Repeat the whole exercise a number of times.

9

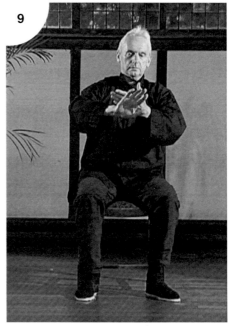

Bring your right hand down in front of your chest with the palm facing out. The palm of your left hand should face your body. Repeat exercise stretching the other way as often as is comfortable.

10

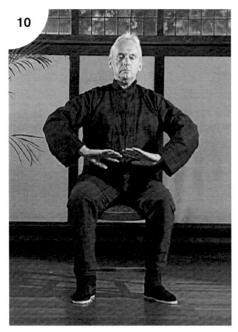

For the last part, bring both hands to your lower abdomen, palms facing away. Breathe in.

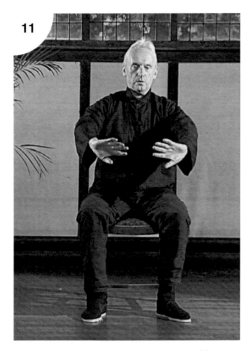

11

While breathing out, press away with both hands.

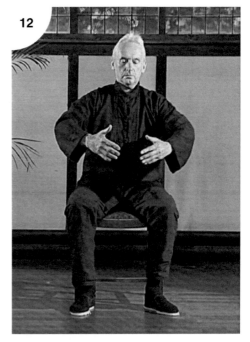

12

Turn your palms up at the end of the breath and, while breathing in, bring your hands back towards your abdomen. Relax your arms at the end. Repeat this a few times.

Remember what we said earlier. You can also do the exercises in Section One standing, but only when you feel comfortable with them.

Do not attempt any of these exercises standing unless you have both feet firmly on they ground.

Take your time; don't rush it.

Section Two
The Next Stage

Once you feel really comfortable with the exercises in Section One, move onto the enhanced exercises in Section Two. Add these new exercises to those you've already learned. You can now become more adventurous. Above all, enjoy yourself.

2.1 Alternative Hand Exercise

This exercise should be done in conjunction with the other hand exercises. It is very strong and the hand exercises in Section One will provide a useful warm up for this one.

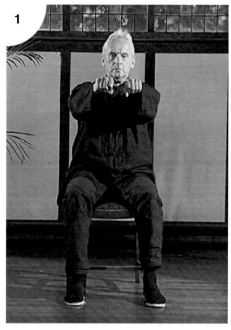

Put your arms out in front of your body with your hands making a soft fist, palms facing down.

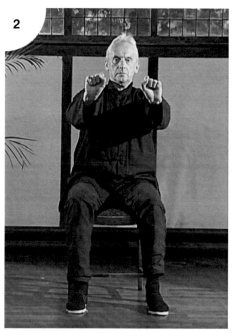

From your wrists, raise both fists up keeping your arms steady. The wrists are making the movement.

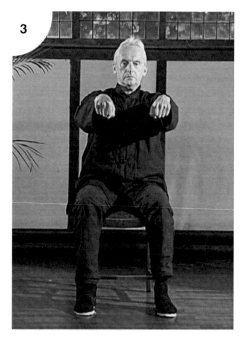

Now drop your wrists down so that your knuckles are facing the floor.

4

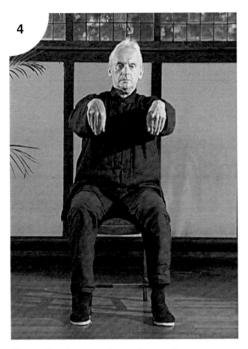

Open the fists and point your fingers down, stretching them as much as is comfortable.

5

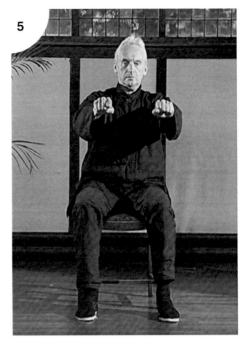

Finally, bring your hands back to the start position. Relax your arms and hands. Repeat this a number of times.

2.2 Tapping

Tiredness or overeating can restrict your blood flow. If you wish to give yourself a short term boost, this exercise will do the trick by transferring blood from the organs and the core of your body to your muscles and nerves. If you are wearing spectacles, please take them off for safety. Complete as much of this exercise as you can.

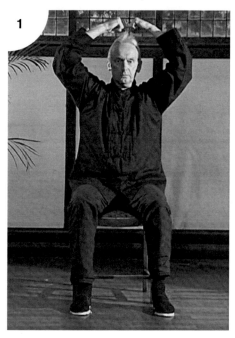

Bring your hands up over your head. You can either have soft, closed fists or leave your palms open.

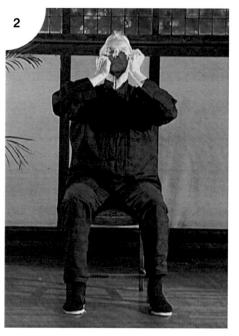

Gently but firmly, start to tap the top of your head using your hands alternately and develop a rhythm. After 10 or 12 taps, transfer the tapping to your forehead; next to your face.

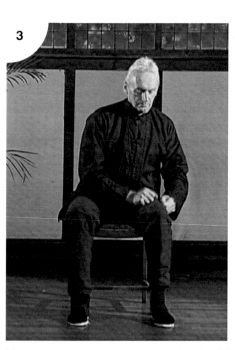

Now move to your jaw, your neck, shoulders, your chest, abdomen then down your leg, back up your leg, down the other leg and back up your body the way you came. Take a small diversion to tap your kidneys.

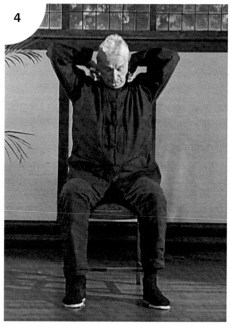

When you return to the top of your head, reach behind to tap the back of your head, neck and back of your shoulders, but only if you're comfortable reaching that far.

Don't worry if you can't reach every part. An ideal exercise would be to complete the all-over routine three times. Don't forget to replace your spectacles. You know what happens when you leave them lying around. Either you lose them or someone stands on them. Neither eventuality is likely to improve your day.

2.3 Extra Breathing

Babies start their breathing cycle from their abdomens. As we age, the stresses of life inhibit this relaxed breathing pattern. We breathe further and further up the abdomen using less and less of our lungs. Over time, the bottoms of our lungs become inactive and stale air becomes trapped.

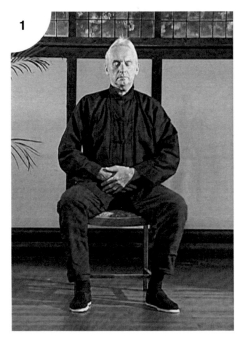

1

Place one hand over the other on your lower abdomen. Gently fill your lungs with air, inhaling through your nose, putting your awareness into your abdomen. Feel your abdomen pushing out as your lungs fill, pushing your hands out. Hold your breath briefly and then allow the air to escape. Allow your hands to move with the inflating and deflating abdomen. Relax briefly at the end of the cycle then start the cycle again.

Complete as many cycles as are comfortable.

Try to practise this exercise in your daily life as you go about your activities. It will soon become a habit and second nature.

2.4 Drawing the Bow

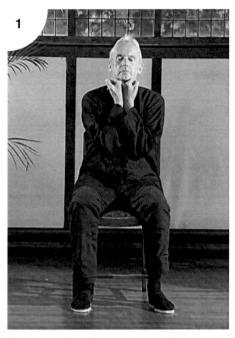

Bring both hands up to your chest, making two soft fists, back to back.

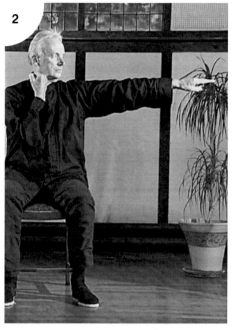

Move your left arm out to the side, straight at shoulder height. The back of your hand should face up with your index and middle fingers pointing straight out, the other fingers curled into the palm.

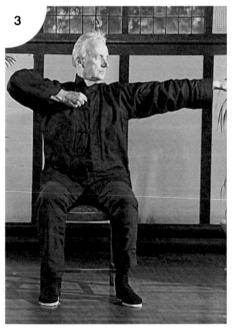

Move your right elbow up bending it at the same time. Leave the fist in place with your palms facing down; fingers facing the floor.

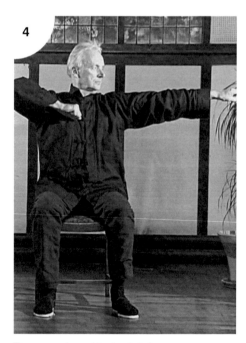

Turn your head to look left as you straighten yor left arm. Head up. Breathe deeply as you make the move. Visualise that you're stretching the bow. Go on. Stretch your arms.

5

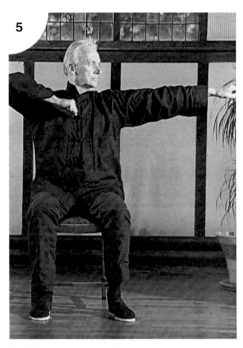

Pull the bowstring tight.

6

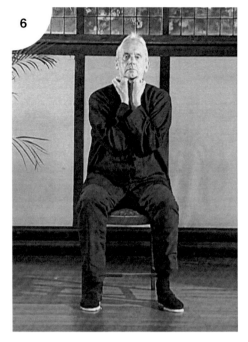

Return to face the front, placing the backs of your fists together. Repeat a few times.

7

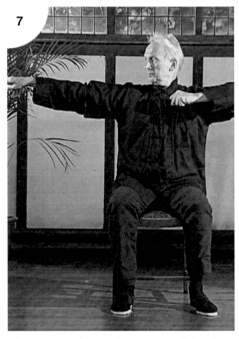

Now repeat the routine on your right side.

Don't worry if you don't make the move correctly. The point is to open the chest and breathe well.

2.5 Vertical Stretch

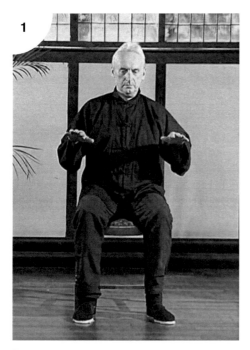

Bring both hands up to your sides keeping your elbows bent; left palm facing up, right palm facing down.

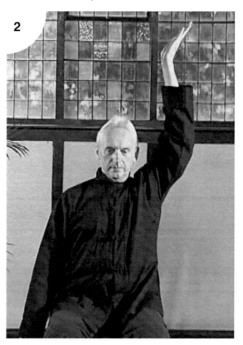

Move your left hand and arm up and, at the same time, move your right arm as far down as possible.

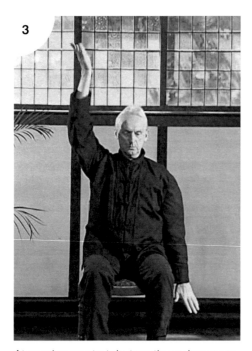

At maximum stretch, turn the palms over and return.

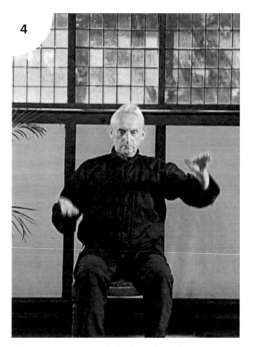

Now move your right hand and arm up and, at the same time, move your left arm as far down as possible. Repeat the movement a number of times. At the end relax your arms. Do this exercise rhythmically and slowly, perhaps 8 or 10 times.

This helps with your co-ordination.

2.6 Opening the Gate

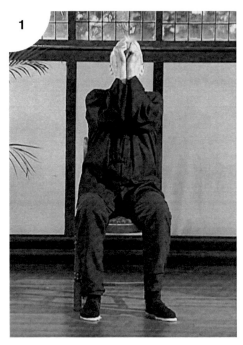

Bring both arms up in front of your body, your hands making fists, finger sides together. Your fists will now be in front of your face.

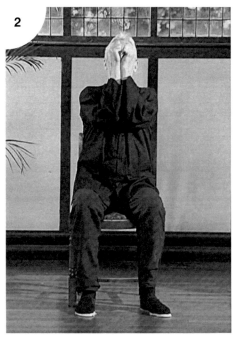

Bring your elbows together, or as close together as you can. Your lower arms should be vertical to the floor.

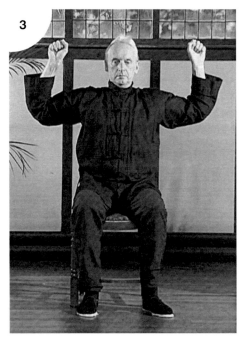

Open both arms outward to the side. At the same time, breathe in.

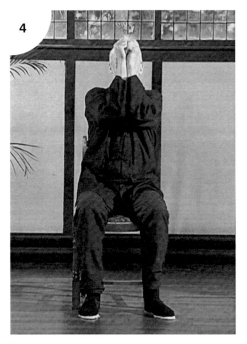

Then bring both arms back to the centre while breathing out. At the completion of this exercise, relax your arms. Repeat this 10 or 12 times.

2.7 Hip Exercise

Treat this exercise with respect. It is especially important to attempt this only if you are in reasonably good health and have a certain amount of movement in these joints.

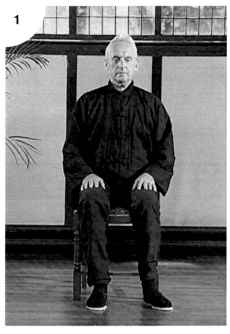

Sit in an upright position with your feet flat on the floor, hands on knees.

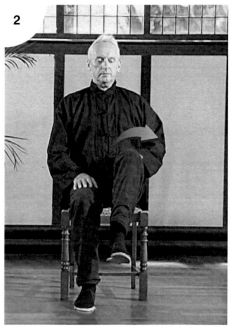

Bring your left leg up keeping it bent.

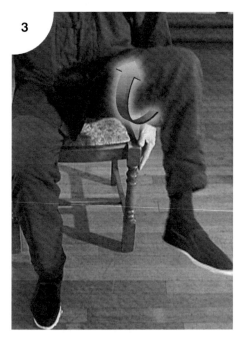

Move it in a slow circle to the left, working from the hip. Move it as slowly as you can and make as big a circle as is comfortable. Try this 1 to 3 times depending on your strength and flexibility.

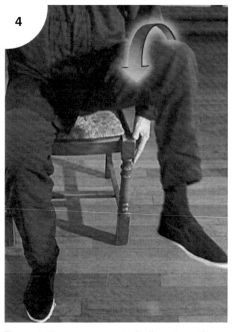

Repeat the movement circling the other way.

5

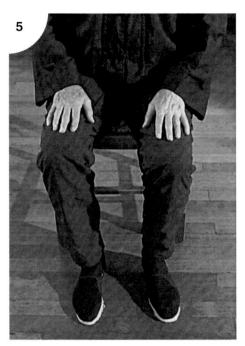

Place your leg back on the floor.

6

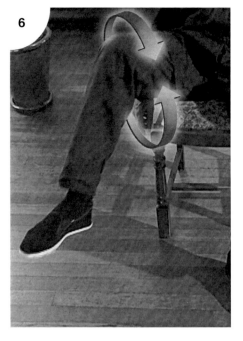

Repeat this exercise with your right leg.

This improves the flexibility of your hips.

Like Section One, when you are comfortable with Section Two's exercises you may wish to do them while standing.

Don't forget the correct stance and be sure you are comfortable with the exercises in Section Three first.

Section Three
Standing Exercises

It is important to work with the standing exercises in order to maintain mobility and independence. Clive always tells his students that he has two objectives in his classes. One is to keep students out of the doctor's surgery and two, to keep them in their homes for as long as possible.

Master Lam, a well known Chinese *chi gong* teacher and writer, says that our legs and our ability to walk well, are direct indicators of our mental and physical health. They are direct indicators of our well-being.

Problems with the legs can be an early sign of ageing and a decline in health.

It is important, as with all these exercises, to make haste slowly. Start with two or three exercises in Section Three and slowly build up. This will greatly enhance your strength, flexibility and stamina.

3.1 The Start Stance

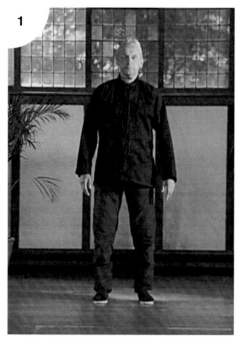

Stand with your feet shoulder-width apart. Point your toes forwards, knees relaxed and bent, shoulders, arms and hands relaxed, back straight, tailbone tucked in, head up and eyes looking forwards.

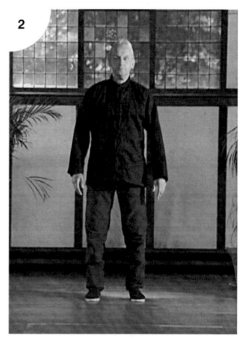

This is an energetic posture in its own right. Energy will flow around the body when in this stance. The weight of the body will drop to the floor through your feet, thereby relieving pressure on your shoulders and lower back. Practising this daily will greatly strengthen your body below the waist.

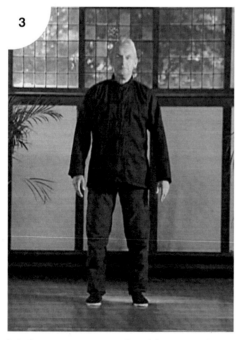

It is important to practise this stance in order to retain the ability to stand. Clive tells of one of his students who travels to his class by bus. As he waits at the bus stop he practises the stance. Any idea how old the student is? No? OK, we'll tell you. He's 80.

All the exercises in Section Three commence with the stance.

3.2 Hand Swinging

This exercise has been practised in China for many generations. It is well known for increasing physical strength as well as building up the immune system. Keep your neck, face and mind relaxed throughout.

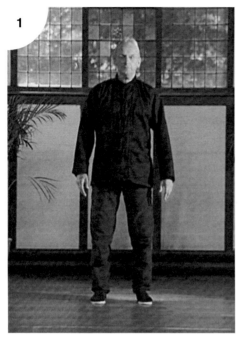

From the start stance keep your shoulders and arms loose and create some space in your armpits.

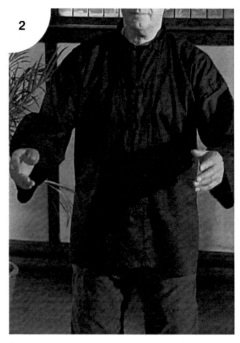

Relax your elbows and fingers. Start to swing your arms forwards and backwards in unison.

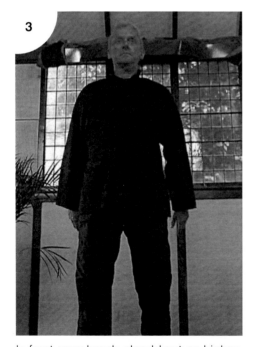

In front, your hands should not go higher than your navel, and the backswing shouldn't pass your buttocks. Swing for as long as is comfortable. Don't overdo this exercise.

3.3 Hip Movement

Don't forget your opening stance. Oh, good. You remembered.

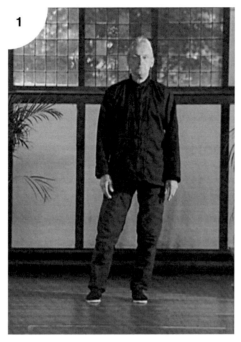

Gently move your left hip outwards keeping your torso straight. Bend your left knee to accommodate the increased weight.

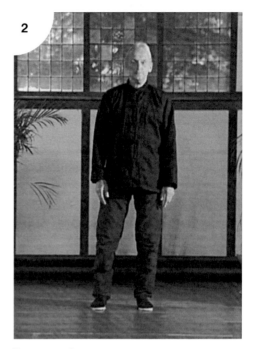

Return to the centre.

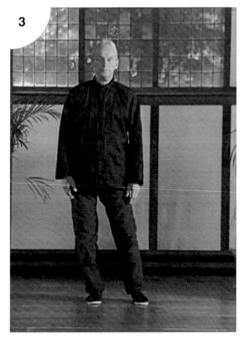

Switch on the right hip, bending your right leg. Repeat a number of times.

This improves flexibility in the hips and strengthens the legs.

3.4 Hip Rotation

Remember the hula hoop? Well, this is a much gentler version.

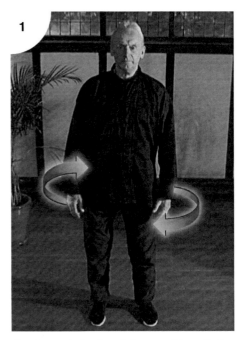

Gently and slowly rotate your hips, first one way, then the other. Make the circles slow and rhythmic and make them small in circumference.

Do maybe 12 or 14 each way.

This is excellent for gently massaging the organs in your lower abdomen as well as exercising your hips, lower spine, ligaments and tendons in your abdomen.

3.5 Side Stretch

The origin of this exercise is Pilates. It is very good for stretching the sides of your body and the tops of your hips.

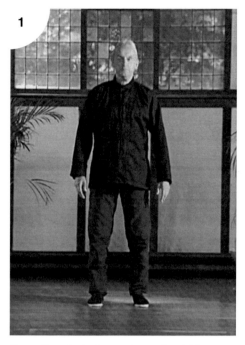

From the start stance (you should be getting used to this now,) relax your left arm down by your side.

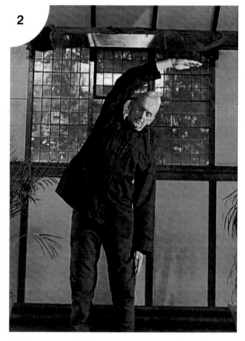

Raise your right arm over your head, palm down, so that the arm and hand make a semi-circle. Feel the side of your body gently stretching as your arm moves up and round. Complete a number of stretches as long as you are comfortable.

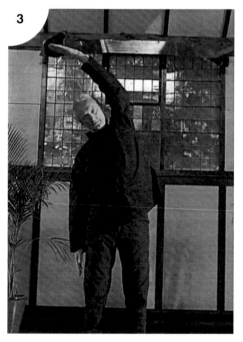

Gently lower the arm and repeat on the other side.

3.6 Leg Strengthening 1

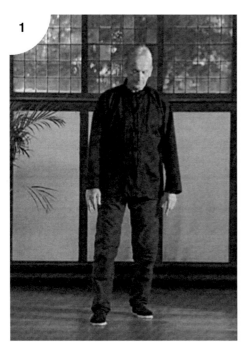

Toes facing forwards, place your right leg in front of your left leg. Your left foot should be at approximately 45° to your right foot. Your feet will be shoulder-width apart. Your torso straight, pointing forward, arms relaxed, knees bent.

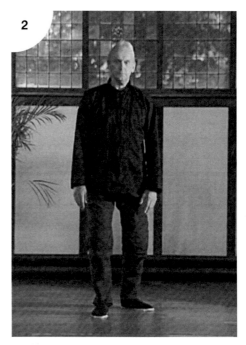

Push your body forward onto your right leg, remembering to keep your torso straight, and bend the weight-bearing knee more. Your right knee should go no further forward than your big toe.

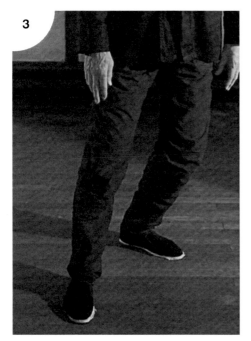

Push back onto your left leg, bending the left knee more to take the weight. Repeat this as many times as is comfortable.

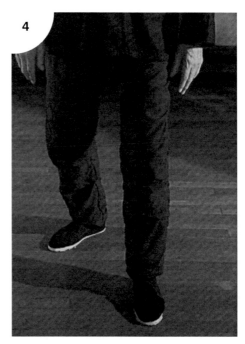

Now change to the other side. Put your left leg forward and right leg at 45°. Repeat the exercise. Keep your torso straight and keep your feet flat on the floor throughout. Develop a relaxed rhythmic action.

3.7 Leg Strengthening 2

Use the same leg movements as Exercise 3.6 above.

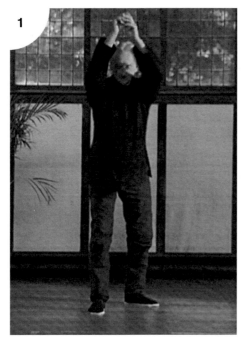

Let your arms swing forward in unison as your front knee bends forward.

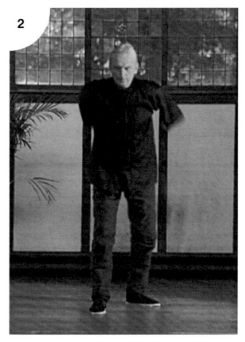

Bring the arms back as the movement returns to the back leg. Make the movement as strong or relaxed as you feel at the time. Repeat as many times as you like providing you feel comfortable.

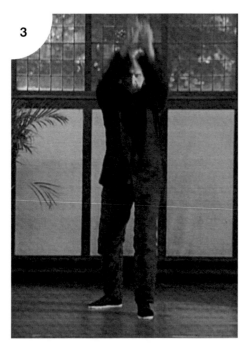

Change sides when you're ready and repeat the exercise.

This exercise is excellent for stress relief and warming up your body.

3.8 Bring Positive Energy into your Body

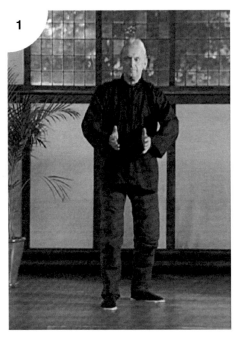

Stay with the leg movements as Exercises 3.6 and 3.7. This time, however, bring both hands in front of your body as if you were holding a ball of energy

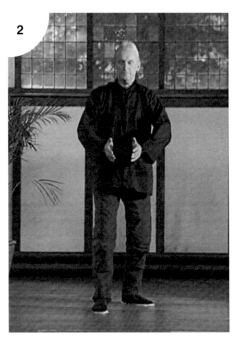

Keep your hands soft, fingers rounded and arms away from your body to keep your armpits free.

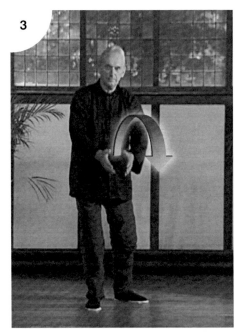

Push your hands down, away and up in a circular motion in unison with the leg movement you've practised in 3.6. and 3.7.

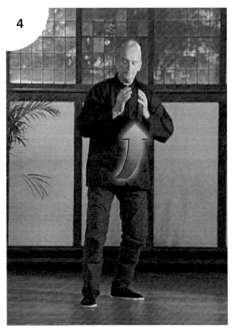

As your hands drop towards your body to complete the circle, drop back onto your rear leg.

5

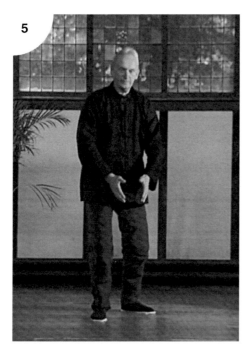

As your hands move away from your body in the circular motion, move onto the forward leg. Make this movement very slowly and rhythmically. Breathe deeply, relax and switch off the thinking process. Repeat the move many times.

6

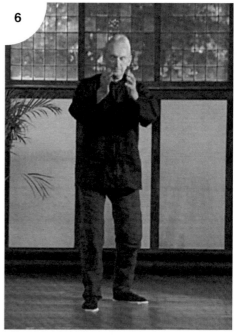

Don't forget to change legs and repeat the exercise.

It is extremely beneficial. It relaxes you and brings *chi* into your body.

3.9 Extra Knee Exercise

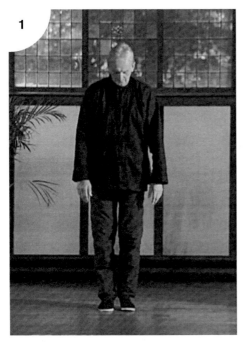

Bring both feet close together. Bend your knees a little more than usual.

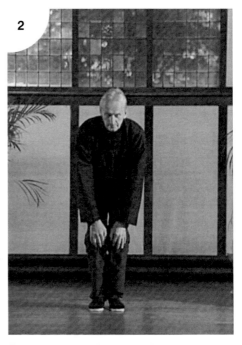

Place both hands on your knees.

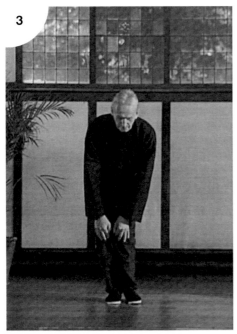

Gently rotate your hands around your knees. Rotate one way then the other. Be careful not to overdo this exercise.

3.10 Lifting the Sky

Both this exercise and Exercise 3.11 are particularly beneficial for inducing energy flow in the body... that's the chi again.

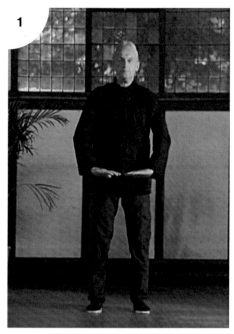

Remembered your start stance? Good. Palms down, place your arms in front as far down your body as possible.

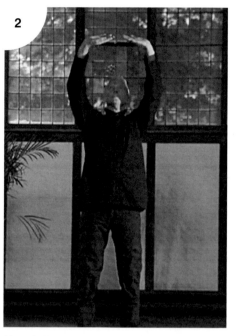

Now bring your arms up in an arc in front of you until they face skyward. Breathe in gently through your nose as you lift your arms.

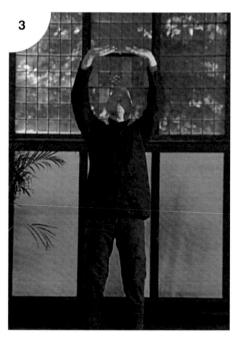

Look up towards your hands and briefly hold your breath.

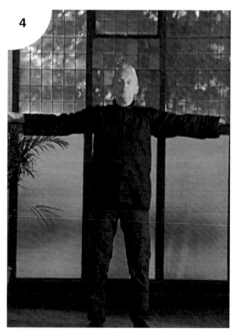

Next, push your arms up and as you gradually straighten your arms, lower them to your sides, gently breathing out as your arms lower. At the same time, feel your back straighten.

5

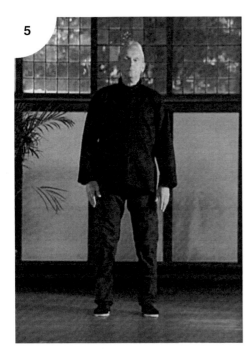

Finally your head returns to its normal position.

6

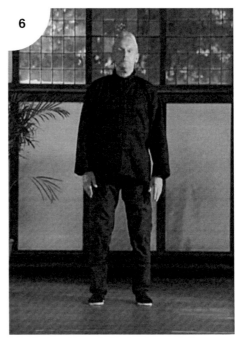

Stand quietly for a few seconds and visualise chi energy flowing from your head down through your body, down your arms and into your fingers, and down your legs to your feet and toes. Initially do this exercise six times.

When you've been doing this exercise for some time you can gradually increase the number of repetitions up to a maximum of twenty.

3.11 Carrying the Moon

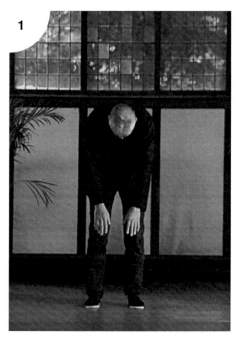

Start stance. Bend your body forward so your arms drop forward effortlessly in front. Make sure your fingers are below knee level. Tuck your head in so that your back forms a continuous curve. As you breathe out, visualise your chi energy flowing up your spine right up to the crown of your head.

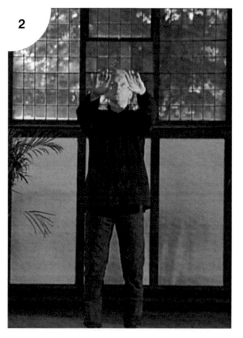

Straighten your body slowly, at the same time lift your arms in a continuous arc to the front, then over your head, all the while breathing in gently.

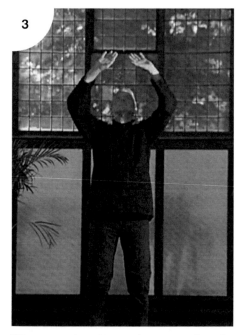

When your hands are above your head, palms up, bend your elbows, separate your thumbs from your fingers as though supporting the curved surface of the moon.

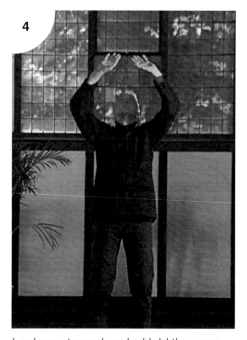

Look up at your hands. Hold the pose and your breath for a few seconds.

5

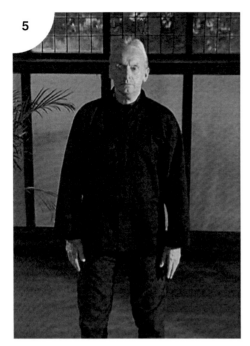

Now straighten your body and lower your arms to your sides, gradually straightening your arms as you do so. Do this while breathing out through your mouth.

6

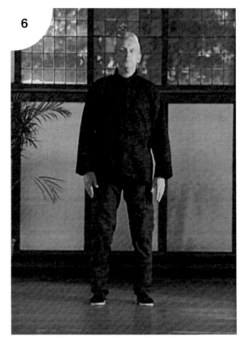

Next, stand quietly for about 30 seconds and visualise chi flowing from your head, down your body, similar to a cascade of water, and on down your arms, fingers, legs, feet and toes. Think of this waterfall as energy, cleansing your body of toxins and negative thoughts. Repeat six times.

As with previous exercises, you can gradually increase the number of repetitions to twenty, if you wish.

In order to extend your flexibility and confidence in standing and walking, remember you can choose to add the exercises from Sections One and Two; standing now, instead of sitting.

Section Four
Eye Movements and Exercises

Eye movements reflect what is happening in consciousness. They are also extremely helpful in developing eyesight. Clive has used this exercise for a number of years and his eyesight has remained constant. His newest pair of spectacles is over ten years old.

Practising these exercises daily will be hugely beneficial.

So, are you ready? Good, let's start.

4.1 Clearing Blockages

This will stimulate the acupuncture points, clear blockages and bring more energy to the eyes.

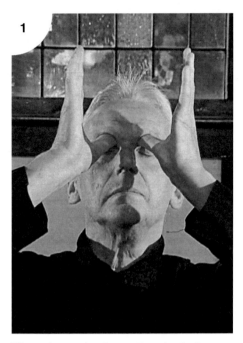

Place the ends of your thumbs in the inner hollow of the eye socket rim at the top of the bridge of your nose. You will feel bumpy bone there. This is the location of acupuncture points, one on each side.

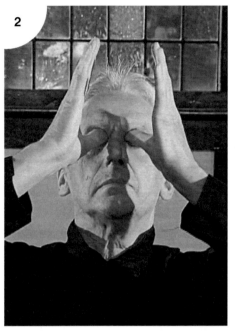

Press the points for around 20 seconds and then gently rotate the thumbs.

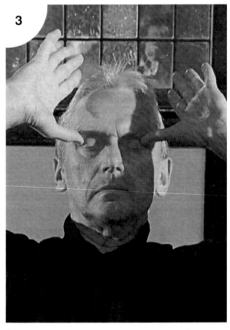

Rotate maybe 10 or 12 times each way.

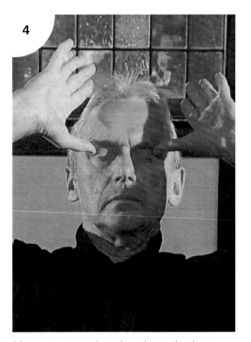

Next, run your thumbs along the bony ridge of the eye socket until you reach halfway above the eye. There you will find two bony protuberances, not as prominent as the first two, but if you concentrate they can be felt. Do the same with the pressure and the rotation as with the first points.

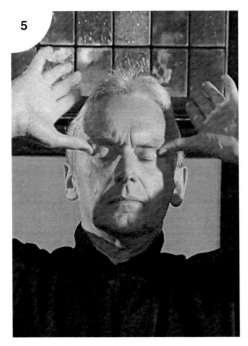

5

Thirdly, run your thumbs to the outer corners of the socket. There are two more bumps there. The indentations are a little less obvious, so be sensitive with your thumb tips. Repeat the pressure and the rotation process.

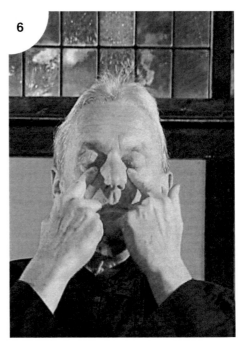

6

Fourthly, place the tips of each of your index fingers halfway along the eye socket and underneath the eye. There are two more indentations there which are also acupuncture points. Repeat the pressure and rotation.

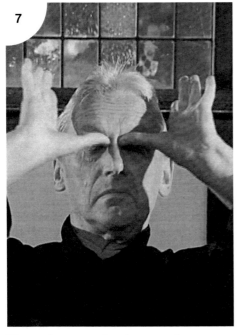

7

The next process involves running your thumbs from the inner hollow near your nose (as in the first exercise) all the way following the line of your eye socket around a far as you can go.

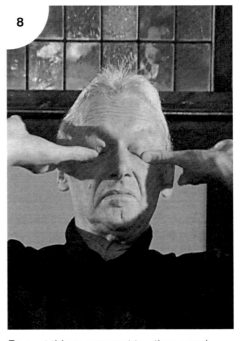

8

Repeat this movement ten times and then ten times the other way; from the bottom of the eye socket near your nose to the start position.

So now we're done

This completes our *chi gong* and other revitalisation exercises. Practise regularly and your health will improve. We hope you enjoy both the exercises and the sense of well-being you will derive from them. Try doing them with your partner or a friend if you can. Make it a social event. This will help make your *chi gong* experience even more enjoyable.